Daddy Loves Me

A color-therapy book for children about their bipolar Daddy

By: GraceMarie Rose

Illustrated by: Zelie Rose

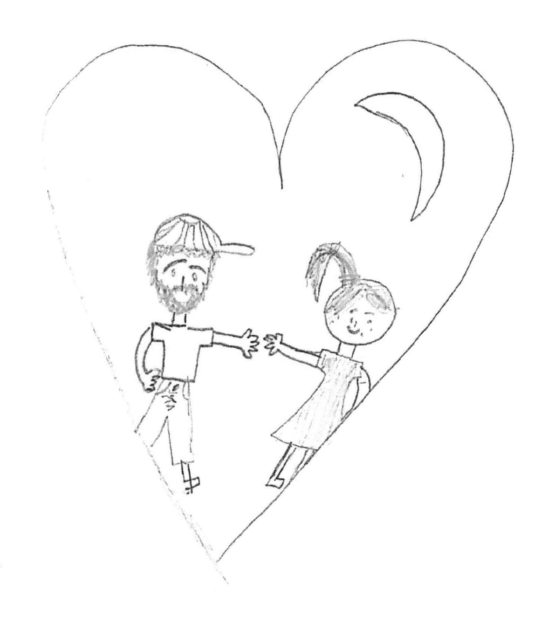

Sometimes Daddy plays with me.

Sometimes Daddy doesn't even see me.

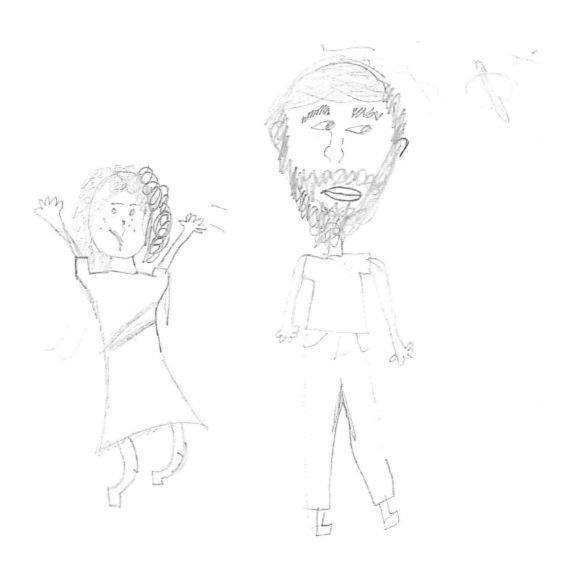

But I know...

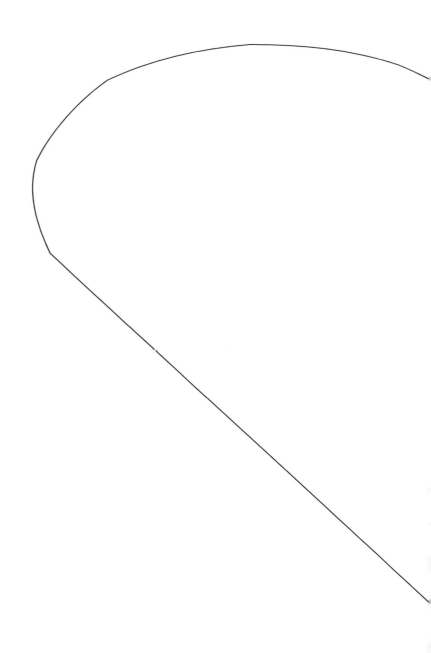

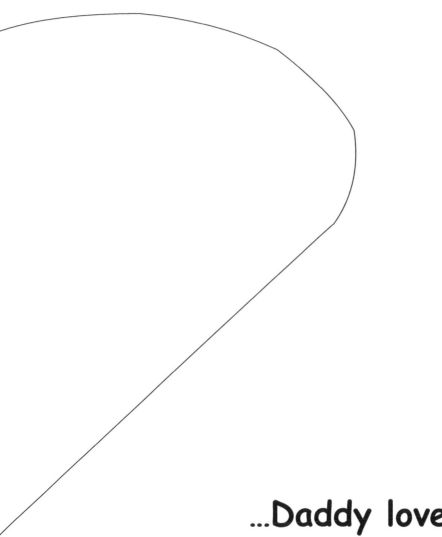

...Daddy loves me.

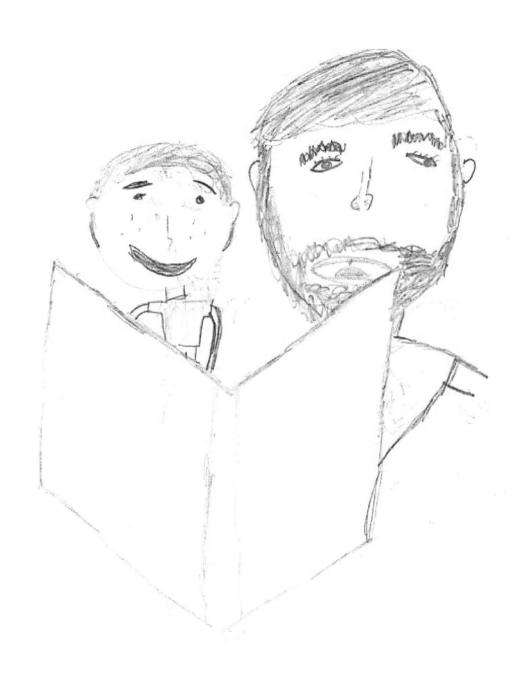

Sometimes Daddy reads me books.

Sometimes Daddy says,
"Leave me alone!"

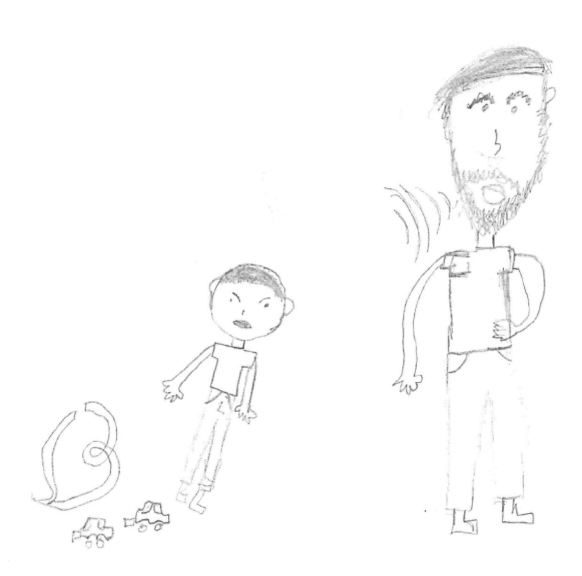

But I know...

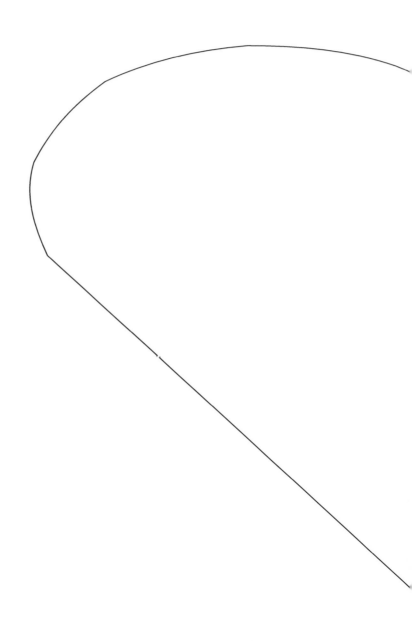

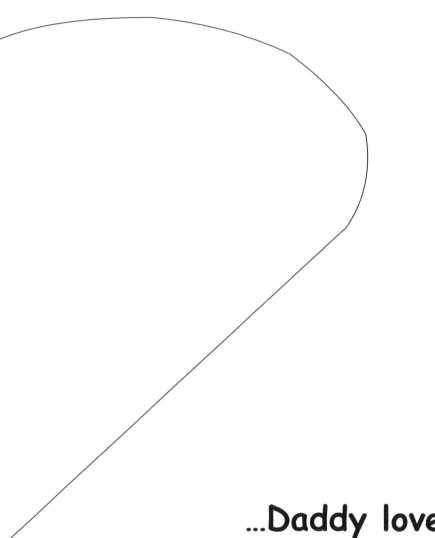

...Daddy loves me.

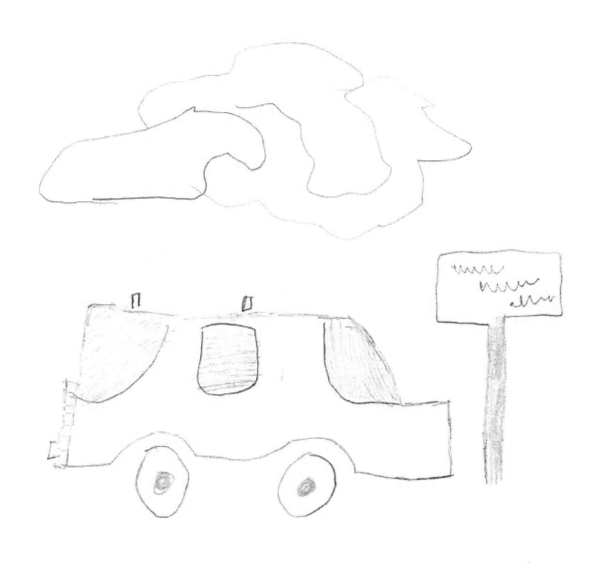

Sometimes Daddy brings me to fun places.

Sometimes Daddy won't come to my game.

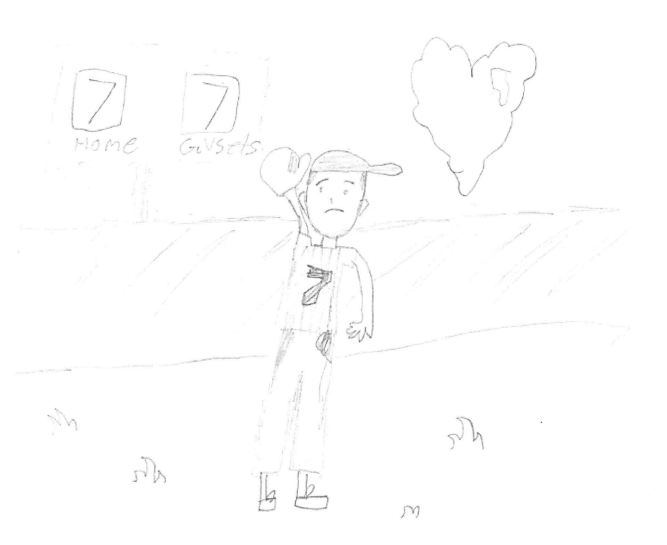

But I know...

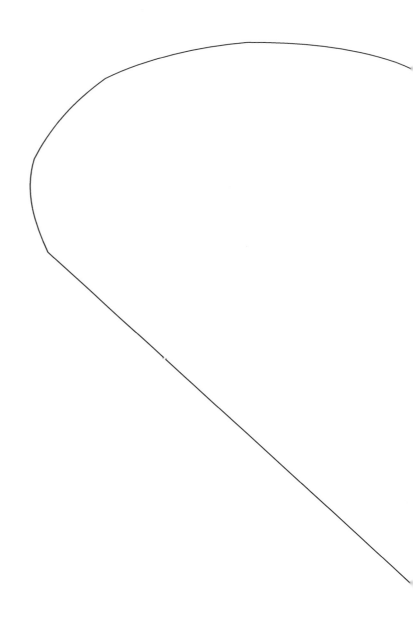

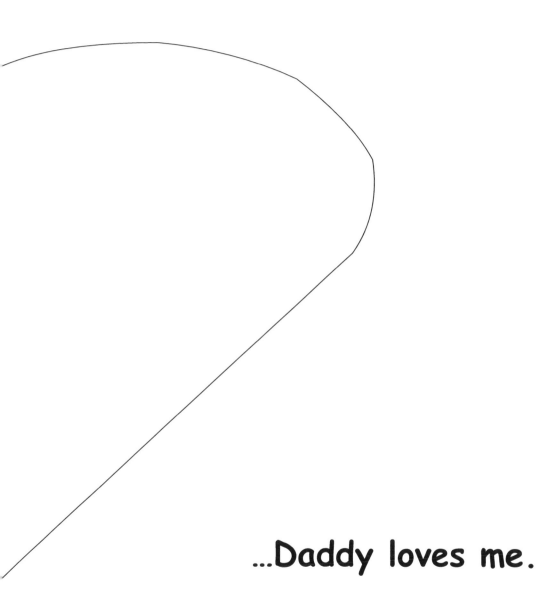

...Daddy loves me.

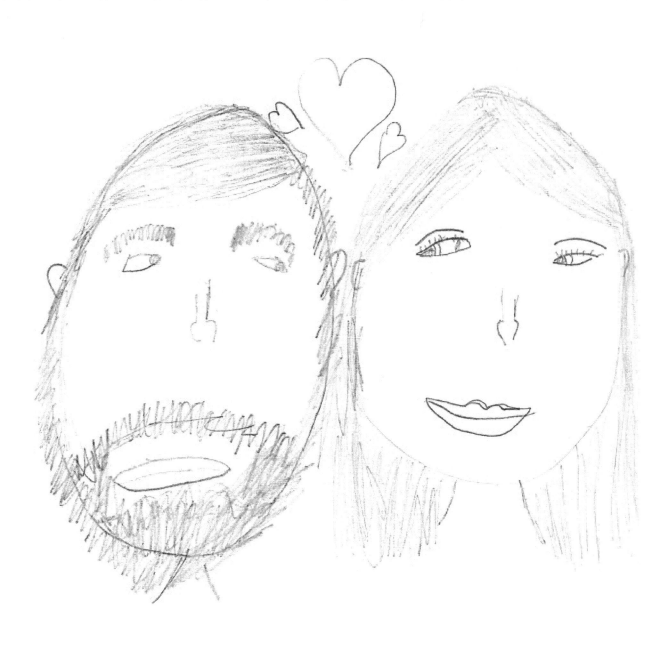

Sometimes Daddy is nice to Mommy.

Sometimes Daddy yells at Mommy.

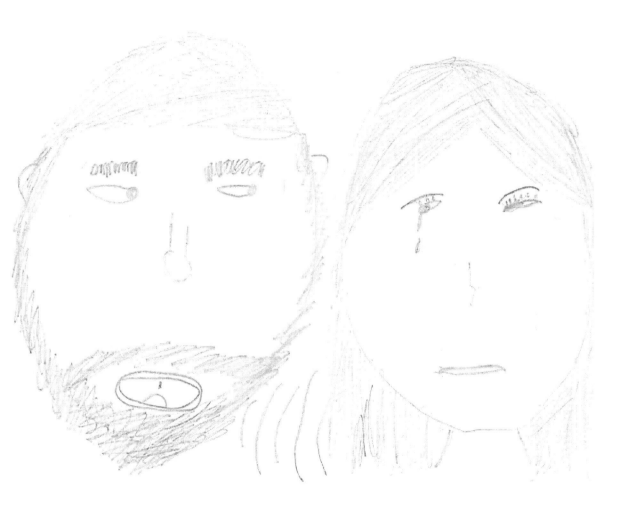

But I know...

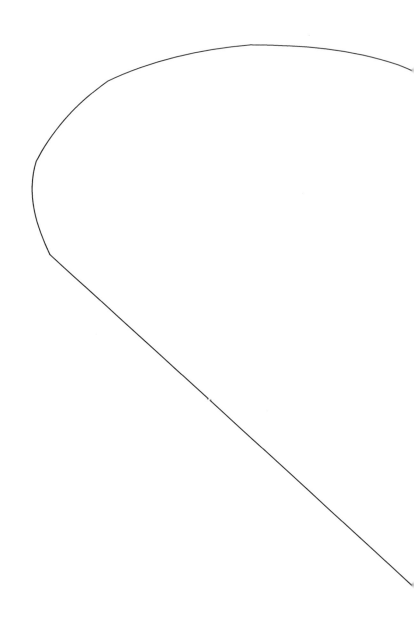

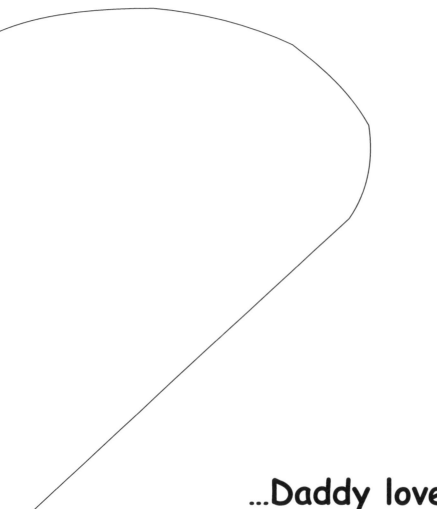

...Daddy loves me.

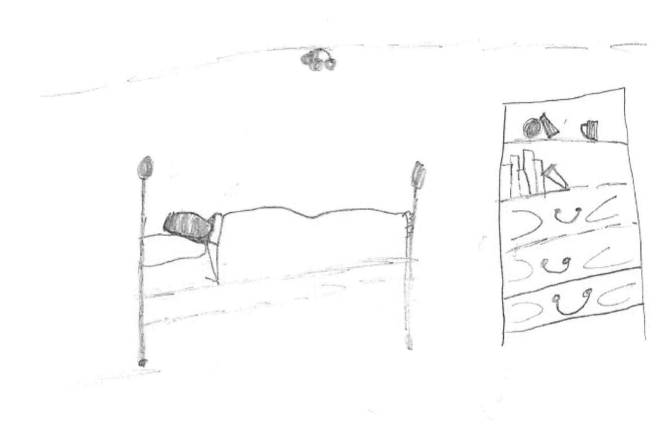

Sometimes Daddy sleeps all day.

Sometimes Daddy goes to the doctor – sometimes for a really long time.

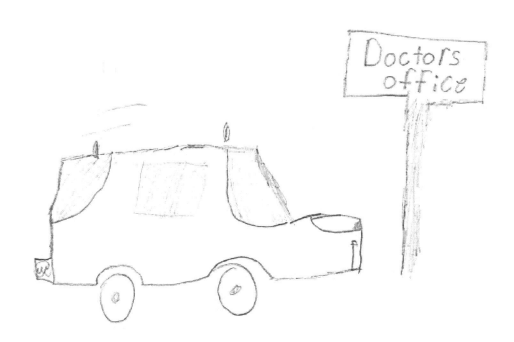

But I know...

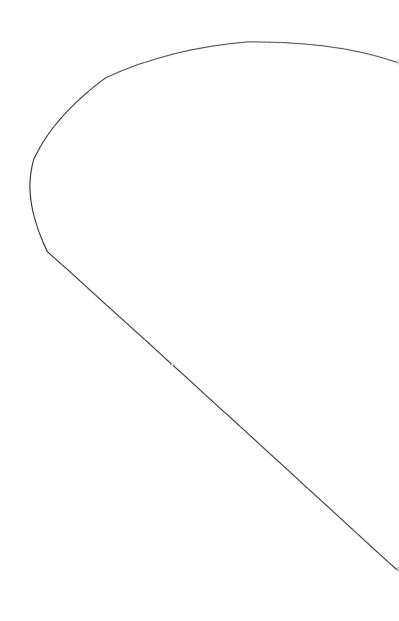

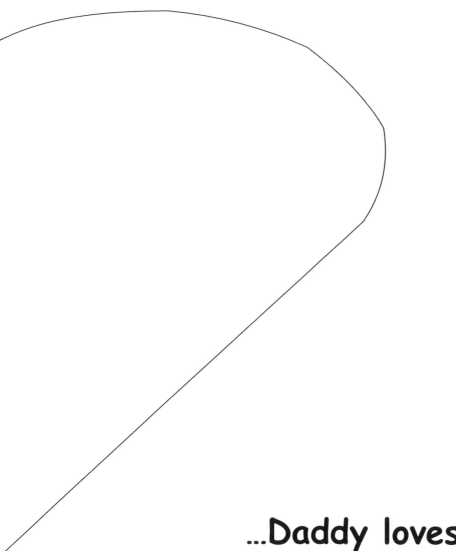

...Daddy loves me.

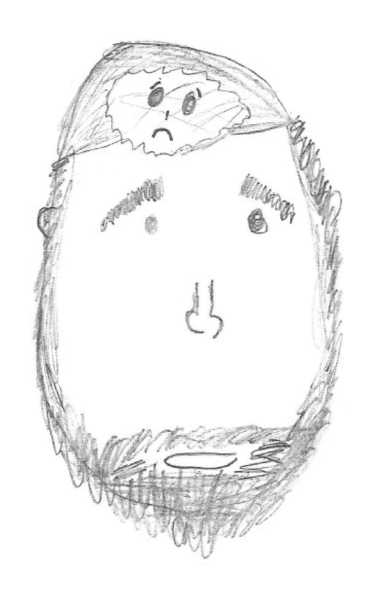

I know that Daddy's brain is sick.

But Daddy's heart is not sick!

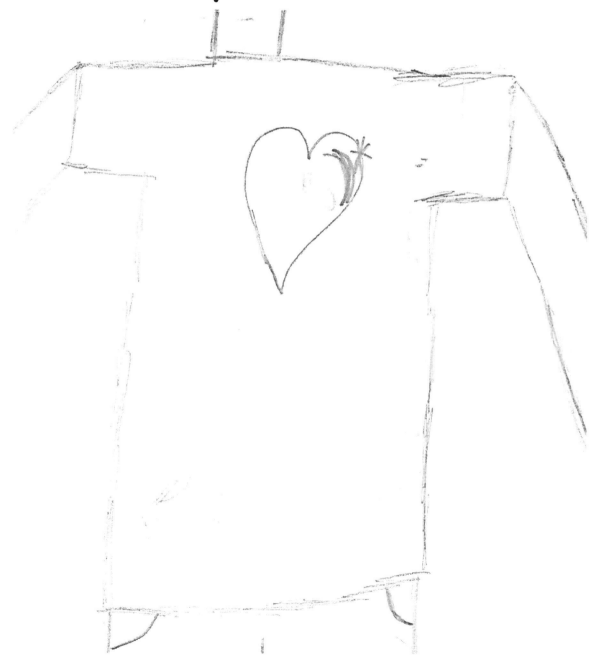

But I know...

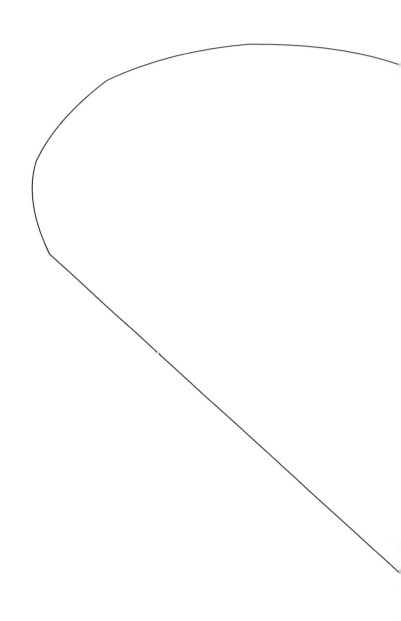

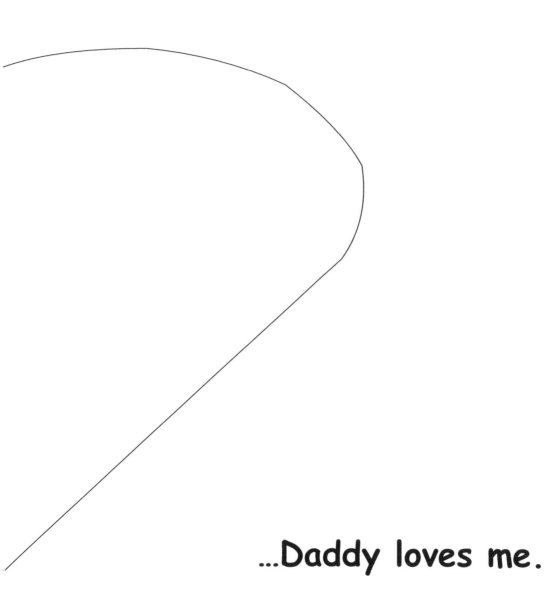

...Daddy loves me.

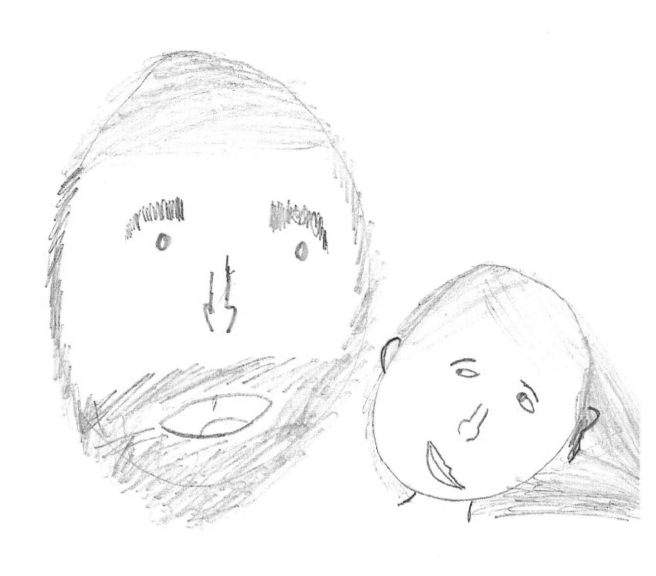

Whether Daddy is with me,

Or living far away,

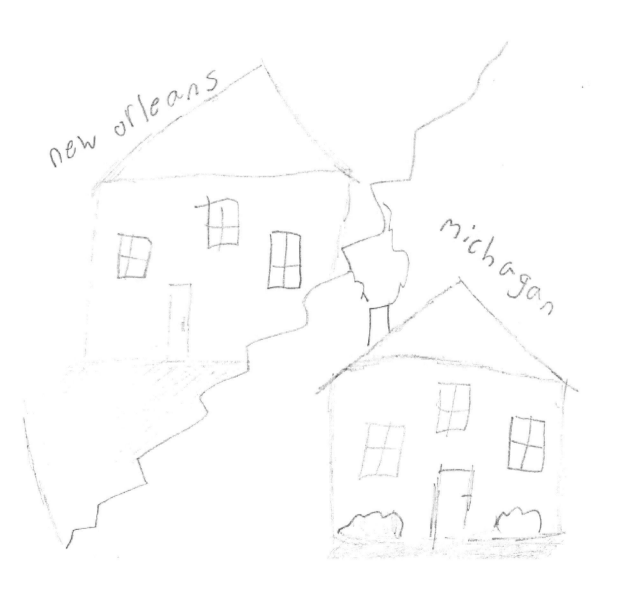

I know...

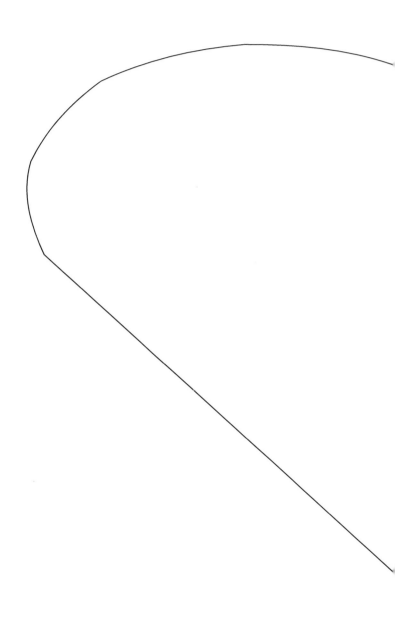

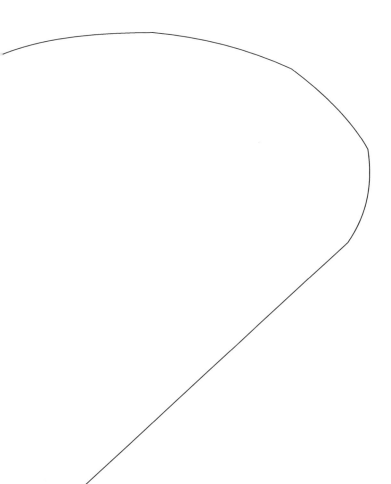

...my Daddy will always love me.